Fibromyalgia Cookbook

Quick & Easy Anti-Inflammatory Recipes for Pain Relief, Fatigue-Fighting, and Physical Recovery

By

SOPHIA PARSON

How to Use This Book

Welcome to the "Fibromyalgia Cookbook" – your ultimate resource for managing fibromyalgia symptoms through the power of nutrition, home exercises, and a 21-day meal plan. Whether you're newly diagnosed or a seasoned warrior in the fight against fibromyalgia, this book is designed to support you on your journey to better health and well-being. Here's how to make the most of it:

Step one: Understand Fibromyalgia

Start by reading the introduction to gain an overview of fibromyalgia, the importance of nutrition, and the purpose of this cookbook. Go to the section on understanding fibromyalgia, where you'll learn about the condition's impact on the body and its symptoms.

Step two: Importance of Nutrition in Managing Fibromyalgia

Dive into the chapter on nutrition, which explores how dietary choices can influence fibromyalgia symptoms and overall health. Explore a variety of recipes specifically crafted to alleviate pain and discomfort associated with fibromyalgia.

Learn about the powerful ingredients that can help reduce inflammation and promote healing in the body.

Step three: 21-Day Meal Plan:

Meal Plans for Fibromyalgia Relief: Discover customizable meal plans tailored to support fibromyalgia management and improve overall well-being. Follow our carefully curated 21-day meal plan designed to provide balanced nutrition while supporting fibromyalgia management.

Step Four: Cooking Techniques and Tips: Find valuable tips and techniques for preparing fibromyalgia-friendly meals with ease and efficiency.

Step Five: Lifestyle Strategies beyond the Kitchen: Explore lifestyle factors such as exercise, stress management, and sleep hygiene that can complement your dietary efforts in managing fibromyalgia.

Step Six: Home Exercises for Physical Recovery: Incorporate gentle yet effective home exercises tailored to support physical recovery and improve mobility.

Step Six: Community and Support:

Connect with others managing fibromyalgia, share experiences, and find support in your journey toward better health.

Step Sven: Conclusion: Wrap up your exploration with a recap of key takeaways and encouragement for continued progress.

Each section of this book is designed to provide you with valuable insights, practical tips, delicious recipes, home exercises, and a structured meal plan to support your fibromyalgia management efforts.

Let this cookbook be your trusted companion on the path to wellness, guiding you toward a life of greater comfort, vitality, and resilience.

TABLE OF CONTENTS

INTRODUCTION

Rose, a once vivacious and exuberant person, became lost in a web of chronic pain, exhaustion, and despair. Determined to reclaim her life, Rose went on a therapeutic path, discovering an unexpected ally in her kitchen - a collection of recipes that would serve as the foundation for her recovery.

Fibromyalgia, which causes widespread musculoskeletal pain, exhaustion, and sleep difficulties, had thrown a pall over Rose's once vibrant life.

She found the transforming impact of nutrition in managing fibromyalgia while looking for alternatives to typical medical treatments.

Nutrition became an important factor in Rose's healing journey. She discovered the power of specific foods to reduce inflammation, boost energy levels, and improve general well-being through meticulous research and advice from healthcare professionals. Rose recognized the importance of nutrition in controlling fibromyalgia and believed that a well-balanced diet might have a significant impact on symptom severity and overall quality of life. Foods high in antioxidants, omega-3 fatty acids, and anti-inflammatory characteristics may alleviate discomfort and help the body manage the complexity of fibromyalgia.

For Rose, this revelation was a watershed moment in her fight against the condition's crippling symptoms.

More than just a collection of recipes, this cookbook envisioned a carefully curated assortment of ingredients to calm, nourish, and uplift.

Each dish is simple, recognizing the limited energy and resources that fibromyalgia patients frequently encounter. From warm soups to nutrient-dense smoothies, the cookbook aims to make the healing process more accessible and pleasurable.

This cookbook is more than a collection of tasty recipes; it is a tool for empowerment. It will enable you to take an active role in controlling your health by recognizing healthful, tasty elements that contribute to your overall well-being.

In a simple terms, the cookbook is a guidebook for navigating the complex relationship between food and fibromyalgia, providing practical suggestions for adopting a diet that nurtures both the body and the mind.

The cookbook is more than just a list of ingredients and directions; it is a companion on the difficult journey to recovery. It reassures you that you are not alone, transforming kitchens into havens of hope and resilience.

This cookbook is more than just a recipe collection; it's an inspiration, reminding people with fibromyalgia that strength can be found in eating nutritious meals, one delicious food at a time.

CHAPTER 1

Understanding Fibromyalgia and Inflammation.

Fibromyalgia is an illness that affects millions of people throughout the world and is similar to a puzzle with illusive components.

Simply put, it shows widespread musculoskeletal discomfort, which is frequently accompanied by exhaustion, sleep disruptions, and cognitive difficulties. While the specific etiology is unknown, genetics, diseases, and physical or mental trauma are thought to contribute to its start.

Fibromyalgia patients frequently have a wide range of symptoms that interfere with their daily life.

Routine activities become a battle against pain and tiredness, necessitating extensive ways to manage and alleviate the difficulties presented by this illness.

The Role of Inflammation in Fibromyalgia

At the heart of the fibromyalgia conundrum is inflammation, which occurs as the body attempts to heal and defend itself. Inflammation is the body's natural response to damage or infection, resulting in the production of chemicals that aid recovery.

However, with fibromyalgia, this defensive system fails. For unknown reasons, the body appears to magnify the inflammatory response, resulting in chronic discomfort and agony.

Consider inflammation as the body's alert system. In fibromyalgia, this system is on high alert, sending pain signals even when there is no obvious damage or infection. This increased inflammation contributes greatly to the pain and sensitivity felt by fibromyalgia patients.

Understanding the function of inflammation in fibromyalgia is critical to developing appropriate therapeutic options. It moves the emphasis from simply treating symptoms to addressing the underlying inflammatory processes. While inflammation is not the only cause, its impact is evident, and focused interventions can help people regain control of their lives.

How Nutrition Influences Inflammation

When it comes to fibromyalgia management, the adage "you are what you eat" takes on new significance. Nutrition is critical in controlling inflammation, providing individuals with a powerful tool to favorably impact their well-being.

Certain foods have anti-inflammatory qualities that help to reduce the heightened immune response associated with fibromyalgia. Consuming a range of antioxidant-rich fruits and vegetables can help to combat oxidative stress and reduce inflammation.

Omega-3 fatty acids, present in fatty fish such as salmon and walnuts, function as natural inflammatory fighters, providing a delightful and healthy method to alleviate fibromyalgia symptoms.

In contrast, processed diets high in sweets and bad fats can aggravate inflammation. These dietary decisions can lead to an imbalance in the gut flora, which has a deleterious impact on the inflammatory response.

Individuals with fibromyalgia who follow a balanced and nutritious diet may be able to alleviate their symptoms and help their bodies manage inflammation more effectively.

CHAPTER 2

Nutritional Foundations for Fibromyalgia Relief

For those navigating the complex landscape of fibromyalgia, understanding the nutritional foundations for treatment becomes a beacon of hope in their quest for well-being.

Beyond drugs and therapy, essential nutrients and a healthy diet emerge as critical components in managing the problems of fibromyalgia.

Essential Nutrients for Fibromyalgia Management

In the quest for fibromyalgia relief, certain nutrients stand out as superheroes, helping to alleviate symptoms and promote overall health.

Vitamin D, also known as the "sunshine vitamin," has shown promise in treating fibromyalgia-related pain and exhaustion. Magnesium, a mineral that regulates muscle function and relaxation, may help relieve muscle cramps and discomfort.

Omega-3 fatty acids, which are abundant in fatty fish like salmon and flaxseeds, have anti-inflammatory effects and provide a natural defense against the heightened inflammation associated with fibromyalgia.

Coenzyme Q10 (CoQ10), an antioxidant, helps to produce cellular energy, which may help to alleviate the persistent exhaustion that fibromyalgia patients suffer.

Ensuring an appropriate intake of these vital nutrients can serve as a starting point for controlling fibromyalgia symptoms, providing a comprehensive approach to alleviation.

Importance of a Balanced Diet.

A well-balanced diet is the foundation of fibromyalgia care, giving the body the skills it needs to deal with the challenges of this condition. Rather than focusing on individual "miracle" foods, nutrition should be approached in a diversified and well-rounded manner.

Incorporating a variety of fruits, vegetables, whole grains, lean meats, and healthy fats ensures a diverse range of nutrients required for good health.

A well-balanced diet not only meets nutritional requirements but also helps with weight management and promotes good musculoskeletal system performance.

This holistic approach promotes resilience, allowing people to better deal with the physical and emotional components of fibromyalgia.

Developing a Fibromyalgia-friendly Kitchen

Turning the kitchen into a fibromyalgia-friendly oasis requires careful planning and deliberate choices.

Stocking up on nutrient-dense foods like colorful veggies, lean proteins, and whole grains helps to create well-balanced meals. Minimizing processed foods, which can cause inflammation, is an important step in building a supportive environment for fibromyalgia management.

Practical methods such as meal planning and kitchen organization can help those suffering from fibromyalgia fatigue. Simplifying cooking processes and choosing simple, nutritious meals make the kitchen a source of sustenance rather than stress.

Recognizing the nutritional basis for fibromyalgia alleviation encourages people to take an active role in their health.

Essential nutrients, a balanced diet, and a fibromyalgia-friendly kitchen all contribute to a complete approach to symptom management and improving overall quality of life for those dealing with fibromyalgia-related issues.

Anti-inflammatory Ingredients

In the search for well-being, investigating anti-inflammatory substances can be a powerful technique for controlling diseases such as fibromyalgia. These components, derived from nature's bounty, can reduce inflammation, providing relief from the ongoing discomfort associated with inflammatory disorders.

Herbs & Spices with Anti-inflammatory Properties

Herbs and spices, which are commonly found in the corners of every kitchen, emerge as unsung heroes in the fight against inflammation.

Turmeric, specifically its main component curcumin, has powerful anti-inflammatory benefits. Ginger, which not only adds zest to foods but also contains gingerol, demonstrates its capacity to reduce inflammation.

Cinnamon, cloves, and rosemary are not only tasty but also anti-inflammatory. Incorporating these herbs and spices into your regular meals not only improves the flavor but also serves as a delightful way to manage inflammation.

Incorporating omega-3 fatty acids

Omega-3 fatty acids, which are well known for their cardiovascular advantages, are also important in reducing inflammation. Fatty fish such as salmon, mackerel, and sardines are high in important fatty acids.

Furthermore, plant-based choices such as flaxseeds, chia seeds, and walnuts provide a vegetarian-friendly method to incorporate omega-3s into your diet.

These fatty acids function as natural inflammation fighters, helping to normalize the body's immunological response. Individuals who include omega-3-rich foods in their daily diets may be able to reduce inflammation and its accompanying symptoms.

Foods Rich in Antioxidants

Antioxidants, the superheroes that fight oxidative stress, are prevalent in a range of foods. Berries, which are colorful and flavorful, are high in antioxidants such as anthocyanins.

Dark leafy greens, such as spinach and kale, contain vitamins and minerals that help the body fight inflammation.

Colorful vegetables, such as bell peppers and tomatoes, as well as fruits like oranges and grapes, contain a wide range of antioxidants. These ingredients not only make meals more vibrant, but they also act together to neutralize free radicals and reduce inflammation.

Incorporating anti-inflammatory components into your everyday diet becomes a tasty and practical way to manage illnesses like fibromyalgia.

Individuals can build a culinary sanctuary by embracing the healing characteristics of herbs, spices, omega-3 fatty acids, and antioxidant-rich foods, which not only tempt the taste sensations but also help the body achieve balance and well-being.

CHAPTER 3

Recipes for Pain Relief

Breakfast Options for Energy and Pain Management

Turmeric-infused Quinoa Breakfast Bowl

Ingredients:

Ingredients:

-1 cup quinoa

-2 cups almond milk.

- One spoonful of turmeric powder.

-1/2 teaspoon cinnamon

- 1/4 cup chopped walnuts or almonds

-1 tablespoon honey or maple syrup.

- Fresh berries for topping.

Preparation:

1. Rinse the quinoa thoroughly before cooking it in almond milk with turmeric and cinnamon.

2. Once cooked, fluff the quinoa with a fork before transferring it to a bowl.

3. Add chopped nuts, honey or maple syrup, and fresh berries.

Servings: Two.

Nutritional benefits: high fiber, protein, and anti-inflammatory effects from turmeric.

Omega-3 Packed Chia Seed Pudding with Berries.

Ingredients:

-1/4 cup chia seeds.

- Add 1 cup almond milk and 1 tablespoon honey or agave syrup.

- 1/2 teaspoon vanilla extract, fresh berries for topping.

Preparation:

1. Combine chia seeds, almond milk, honey, and vanilla essence in a bowl.

2. Refrigerate for at least 4 hours or overnight until thickened.

3. Finish with fresh berries before serving.

Servings: Two.

Nutritional benefits: omega-3 fatty acids, fiber, and antioxidants from berries.

Anti-inflammatory Avocado Toast with Smoked Salmon

Ingredients:

- Two pieces of whole grain bread

- One ripe avocado

- One teaspoon of lemon juice.

- Smoked salmon slices.

- Red pepper flakes (optional).

- Add salt and pepper to taste.

Preparation:

1. Toast the whole grain bread pieces.

2. Mash the ripe avocado and add lemon juice, salt, and pepper.

3. Spread mashed avocado on the toasted bread, then top with smoked salmon.

4. Add red pepper flakes if desired.

Servings: Two.

Nutritional Contents: - fats, salmon has omega-3, and it has anti-inflammatory qualities.

Protein-rich Greek Yogurt Parfait with Almond Butter

Ingredients:

-1 cup Greek yogurt.

- 2 tablespoons almond butter

- 1 tablespoon honey

- granola for topping, and sliced bananas.

Preparation:

1. In a glass, combine the Greek yogurt, almond butter, honey, and granola.

2. Repeat the layers.

3. Before serving, top with banana slices.

Serves: 1

Nutritional Contents: - Greek yogurt provides high protein, almond butter provides healthy fats, and cereal provides energy.

Spinach and Mushroom Egg White Omelette.

Ingredients:

-4 egg whites.

- Use a handful of spinach

- 1/2 cup of chopped mushrooms.

- Add 1 tablespoon olive oil and season with salt and pepper to taste.

Preparation:

1. Cook spinach and mushrooms in olive oil until wilted.

2. Whisk the egg whites and pour over the vegetables.

3. Cook until set, then fold and serve.

Servings: 1

Nutritional contents: Low in fat, high in protein, and packed with vitamins from spinach and mushrooms.

Fiber-rich oatmeal with fresh fruits and nuts.

Ingredients:

- 1 cup of rolled oats

- 2 cups almond milk

- One spoonful of chia seeds

- 1/2 cup mixed fresh fruits (berries and banana slices)

- 2 tablespoons chopped nuts (almonds and walnuts)

- 1 tablespoon of maple syrup or honey.

Preparation:

1. Cook rolled oats in almond milk and add chia seeds.

2. Once cooked, garnish with fresh fruits, and chopped nuts, and drizzle with honey or maple syrup.

Servings: Two.

Nutritional content: high fiber from oats and chia seeds, vitamins from fruits, and healthy fats from almonds.

Salmon & Sweet Potato Hash with Turmeric

Ingredients:

- 1 cup cooked and Iced sweet potatoes

 - 1/2 cup cooked salmon flakes

- One teaspoon of turmeric powder and 1 tablespoon olive oil

- Season with salt and pepper to taste - Garnish with fresh parsley.

Preparation:

1. Sauté sweet potatoes, salmon, and turmeric in olive oil until warm.

2. Season with salt and pepper, then garnish with fresh parsley.

Servings: Two.

Nutrition: - Salmon contains omega-3 fatty acids, turmeric has anti-inflammatory properties, and sweet potatoes include complex carbs.

Green Smoothie Bowl With Kale and Pineapple

Ingredients:

- 2 cups kale leaves with stems removed.

- One cup of pineapple pieces

- One-half banana

- One-half cup almond milk

- One spoonful of chia seeds

- Top with granola and sliced kiwi.

Preparation:

1. Blend the kale, pineapple, banana, and almond milk until smooth.

2. Pour into a bowl and top with chia seeds, granola, and sliced kiwi.

Serves: 1

Nutritional Contents: antioxidants from kale and pineapple, omega-3 from chia seeds, and vitamins from kiwi.

Cinnamon Walnut Buckwheat Pancakes

Ingredients:

- 1 cup buckwheat flour and 1 teaspoon baking powder

- 1/2 teaspoon cinnamon and 1/2 cup chopped walnuts.

- Use 1 cup almond milk and 1 tablespoon coconut oil.

- Maple syrup to drizzle.

Preparation:

1. Combine buckwheat flour, baking powder, cinnamon, and chopped walnuts in a mixing dish.

2. Combine almond milk and coconut oil to make a batter.

3. Cook pancakes on the griddle until golden brown.

4. Drizzle with maple syrup before serving.

Servings: Two.

Nutritional Contents: - Rich in fiber from buckwheat, omega-3 from walnuts, and low in gluten.

Coconut milk and berry quinoa porridge

Ingredients:

- 1 cup cooked quinoa

- 1/2 cup coconut milk.

- Add 1/2 cup mixed berries (strawberries, blueberries) and 2 tablespoons shredded coconut.

- One tablespoon full of honey or agave syrup.

Preparation:

1. Mix cooked quinoa, coconut milk, berries, and shredded coconut.

2. Warm on the burner until thoroughly warm.

3. Drizzle with honey or agave syrup before serving.

Servings: Two.

Nutritional Contents: Quinoa contains protein and fiber, while coconut milk delivers healthy fats and natural sweetness.

Lunches to Boost Physical Recovery

Anti-inflammatory turmeric Chicken Salad

Ingredients:

- 2 boneless, skinless chicken breasts, roasted and sliced

- 1 teaspoon turmeric powder

- Mixed salad greens (spinach, arugula, kale)

- Halved cherry tomatoes

- Sliced cucumber

- Thinly slice 1/4 cup red onion and drizzle with olive oil and lemon dressing.

- Add salt and pepper to taste.

Preparation:

1. Apply turmeric powder to grilled chicken slices.

2. In a bowl, add the mixed greens, cherry tomatoes, cucumber, and red onion.

3. Place the turmeric-infused chicken on top.

4. Drizzle with olive oil and lemon dressing, then season with salt and pepper.

Servings: Two.

Nutritional Contents: Chicken provides lean protein, turmeric offers anti-inflammatory effects, and vegetables provide vitamins.

Omega-3 Packed Salmon Power Bowl

Ingredients:

- 1 cup cooked quinoa.

Serve with grilled or baked salmon, steamed broccoli, and sliced avocado.

- Shredded carrots.

- Sesame seeds as garnish

- Soy-ginger dressing.

Preparation:

1. Place the quinoa in a bowl and top with salmon, broccoli, avocado, and shredded carrots.

2. Drizzle with the soy-ginger dressing and sprinkle with sesame seeds.

Servings: Two.

Nutritional content: omega-3 from salmon, protein from quinoa, and several vitamins from vegetables.

Quinoa and Vegetable Stuffed Bell Peppers.

Ingredients:

- 4 halved bell peppers with seeds removed

- 1 cup cooked quinoa

- Mixed vegetables (bell peppers, zucchini, cherry tomatoes)

- 1/2 cup black beans (drained and rinsed)

- Add 1 teaspoon cumin and 1/2 teaspoon chili powder.

- Salsa for topping.

Preparation:

1. Preheat oven to 375°F (190°C).

2. In a bowl, combine the cooked quinoa, mixed vegetables, black beans, cumin, and chili powder.

3. Fill the bell pepper halves with quinoa mixture.

4. Bake for 25-30 minutes, until the peppers are soft.

5. Garnish with salsa before serving.

Serves: 4

Nutritional content: - Quinoa and black beans provide high fiber and protein, while vegetables provide vitamins.

Ginger and Turmeric Carrot Soup

Ingredients:

- 1 pound peeled and diced carrots

 - 1 onion, chopped - 2 garlic cloves, minced

- Grate 1 tablespoon of fresh ginger.

-Add one spoonful of turmeric powder. .

- 4 cups vegetable broth

- Add salt and pepper to taste

- Garnish with coconut milk

Preparation:

1. Cook onion, garlic, and ginger in a saucepan until softened.

2. Combine the chopped carrots, turmeric, and vegetable broth.

3. Simmer until the carrots are soft.

4. Blend until smooth, then spice up with salt and pepper.

5. Finish with a drizzle of coconut milk.

Serves: 4

Nutritional Contents: Turmeric provides anti-inflammatory effects, carrots contain vitamins, and ginger boosts immunity.

Avocado and Spinach Smoothie with Flaxseeds

Ingredients:

- 1 cup spinach leaves and 1/2 avocado.

- One-half banana

- One spoonful of flaxseeds

- One cup of almond milk and Ice cubes (Optional)

- Honey for sweetness is optional.

Preparation:

1: Blend spinach, avocado, banana, flaxseeds, and almond milk until smooth.

2. If desired, add ice cubes and mix again.

3. If needed, sweeten with honey.

Serves: 1

Nutritional Contents: - Avocado has healthy fats, flaxseeds include omega-3 fatty acids, while spinach and banana provide vitamins.

Mediterranean chickpea salad with olive oil dressing.

Ingredients:

- 1 can (15 oz) drained and rinsed chickpeas

 - 1 cup cherry tomatoes, halved

- 1 cucumber, diced

- 1/2 red onion, finely chopped

- 1/2 cup Kalamata olives, sliced

- 1/2 cup crumbled feta cheese

- Fresh parsley, chopped

- Dressing with olive oil, lemon juice, and garlic

 - Salt and pepper to taste.

Preparation:

1. In a large mixing bowl, add chickpeas, cherry tomatoes, cucumber, red onion, olives, and feta cheese.

2. To make the dressing, combine olive oil, lemon juice, and minced garlic in a small bowl.

3. Pour the dressing over the salad and gently stir.

4. Add salt and pepper to taste.

5. Sprinkle with fresh parsley before serving.

Serves: 4

Nutritional content: - Chickpeas are high in fiber and plant-based protein, while olives and olive oil provide healthful fats and vitamins.

Baked sweet potatoes with cinnamon and coconut oil.

Ingredients:

- Scrub and pierce 2 sweet potatoes with a fork

- Melt 1 tablespoon coconut oil

 - Sprinkle 1 teaspoon cinnamon

- Add a pinch of sea salt - Optional: Top with Greek yogurt

Preparation:

 1. Preheat oven to 400°F (200°C).

2. Season sweet potatoes with melted coconut oil, cinnamon, and a pinch of sea salt.

3. Bake for 45-60 minutes, or until soft.

4. Add a dollop of Greek yogurt if preferred.

Servings: Two.

Nutritional Contents: - Sweet potatoes provide beta-carotene, coconut oil contains healthy fats, and cinnamon adds flavor.

Berry Blast Chia Seed Pudding.

Ingredients:

-1/4 cup chia seeds.

- Add 1 cup almond milk and 1/2 cup mixed berries (strawberries, blueberries, raspberries).

- One teaspoon full of honey or agave syrup

- Almond slices for topping.

Preparation: 1. mix chia almond and seeds milk in a bowl.

2. Refrigerate for at least 4 hours or overnight until thickened.

3. Top the chia pudding with mixed berries.

4. Drizzle with honey or agave syrup, then top with almond pieces.

Servings: Two.

Nutritional Contents: - High in omega-3 fatty acids from chia seeds, antioxidants from berries, and naturally delicious.

Green Tea-Infused Quinoa Bowl with Grilled Chicken

Ingredients:

- 1 cup cooked quinoa

- 2 grilled chicken breasts (sliced)

-1 cup steamed broccoli

-1 tablespoon green tea leaves (matcha), and sesame seeds for decoration.

- Soy sauce and ginger dressing.

Preparation:

1. Infuse hot, cooked quinoa with green tea leaves.

2. Place the quinoa in a bowl and top with grilled chicken and cooked broccoli.

3. Drizzle with the soy sauce-ginger dressing.

4. Garnish with sesame seeds.

Servings: Two.

Nutritional content: high protein from chicken and quinoa, antioxidants from green tea, and vitamins from broccoli.

Antioxidant-Rich Berry and Kale Smoothie

Ingredients:

- 1 cup kale greens with stems removed

- 1/2 cup mixed berries (blueberries and strawberries)

- One-half banana and one spoonful of chia seeds

- One cup of almond milk and Ice cubes (Optional)

- Maple syrup for sweetness (optional).

Preparation:

1. Blend the kale, mixed berries, banana, chia seeds, and almond milk until smooth.

2. If desired, add ice cubes and mix again.

3. If needed, sweeten with maple syrup.

Serves: 1

Nutritional content: - Rich in antioxidants from berries and kale, omega-3 from chia seeds, and vitamins from kale and berries.

NOURISHING DINNERS

Turmeric-infused Quinoa Bowl with Roasted Vegetables

Ingredients:

- 1 cup washed quinoa.

- 2 cups vegetable broth and 1 teaspoon turmeric powder.

- 1 teaspoon turmeric powder

- Assorted vegetables (e.g., bell peppers, zucchini, cherry tomatoes)

- 2 tablespoons olive oil

- Salt and pepper to taste

- Fresh cilantro for garnish

Preparation:

1. Cook quinoa in vegetable broth with turmeric powder to package instructions.

2. Toss various vegetables with olive oil, salt, and pepper.

3. Roast the vegetables until they are soft.

4. Place the quinoa in bowls, top with roasted vegetables, and garnish with fresh cilantro.

Servings: Two.

Nutritional Contents: - Quinoa provides high fiber and protein, turmeric has anti-inflammatory properties, and vegetables contain a variety of vitamins.

Salmon and Avocado Citrus Salad with Mixed Greens.

Ingredients: -

 Grilled or baked salmon fillets

 - Mixed salad greens (such as spinach, arugula, or kale)

- one avocado, sliced

- one grapefruit, segmented

- One orange, segmented

- Two tablespoons of balsamic vinaigrette.

- Add salt and pepper to taste.

Preparation:

1. Arrange the mixed greens on a platter.

2. Add grilled or baked salmon, sliced avocado, grapefruit, and orange segments.

3. Drizzle with balsamic vinaigrette, then season with salt and pepper.

Servings: Two.

Nutritional contents: omega-3 from salmon, good fats from avocado, and vitamin C from citrus fruits.

Ginger and turmeric chicken soup with quinoa and kale.

Ingredients:

- 1 pound diced boneless

- skinless chicken breasts

- 1 cup rinsed quinoa

- 1 bunch chopped kale

- 1 onion diced

- 3 sliced carrots

- 3 sliced celery stalks

- 2 minced garlic cloves

- 1 tablespoon grated fresh ginger

- 1 teaspoon turmeric powder.

- 8 cups chicken broth - Add salt and pepper to taste - Serve with fresh lemon wedges.

Preparation:

1. Cook onion, garlic, and ginger in a large pot until softened.

2. Add the diced chicken and heat until browned.

3. Mix in the quinoa, carrots, celery, and turmeric powder.

4. Pour in the chicken broth and heat to a boil.

5. Reduce the heat, add the greens, and cook until the quinoa is done.

6. Season with salt and pepper.

7. Serve hot, with fresh lemon slices on the side.

Serves: 4

Nutritional Contents: - Chicken and quinoa provide protein, turmeric provides anti-inflammatory effects, while kale and veggies contain vitamins.

Baked cod with lemon and herb quinoa pilaf.

Ingredients:

- 2 cod fillets

-1 cup rinsed quinoa

- 2 cups vegetable broth, and 1 lemon zest and juice.

- Chop fresh herbs (e.g., parsley, dill) \- Add olive oil.

- Add salt and pepper to taste.

- Serve with lemon wedges.

Preparation:

1. Preheat oven to 400°F (200°C).

2. Spice up the cod fillets with salt, pepper, and a drizzle of olive oil.

3. Bake the cod in the oven for 15-20 minutes, or until thoroughly done.

4. In a pot, boil the quinoa in vegetable broth until frothy.

5. Fluff quinoa with a fork, then stir in lemon zest, juice, and fresh herbs.

6. Serve cooked cod over a bed of lemon and herb quinoa pilaf.

7. Garnish with more herbs and serve with lemon wedges.

Servings: Two.

Nutritional Contents: - Rich in lean protein from fish, fiber and protein from quinoa, and vitamins from fresh herbs and lemon.

Spinach and Chickpea Curry with Basmati Rice.

Ingredients:

- Drain and rinse 1 can (15 oz) chickpeas

- Finely chop 1 onion

- Mince 2 cloves garlic

- Grate 1 tablespoon fresh ginger

- Two cups of fresh spinach leaves

-One can (14 oz) of diced tomatoes

- One can (14 ounces) coconut milk

- Two tablespoons of curry powder.

- 1 teaspoon cumin

- Salt and pepper to taste

- Cooked basmati rice for serving

Preparation:

1. Cook onion, garlic, and ginger in a saucepan until softened.

2. Combine the chickpeas, spinach, diced tomatoes, coconut milk, curry powder, and cumin.

3. Simmer until the spinach wilts and the flavors blend.

4. Add salt and pepper to taste.

5. Serve with cooked basmati rice.

Serves: 4

Nutritional Contents: - Chickpeas and spinach provide high fiber and plant-based protein, while fragrant spices add to taste.

Grilled turkey breast with sweet potato mash and asparagus.

Ingredients:

-2 turkey breast fillets

- 2 peeled and chopped sweet potatoes, and 1 trimmed bunch of asparagus.

- 2 tablespoons olive oil

- 1 teaspoon dried thyme

- salt and pepper to taste

- fresh parsley for garnish.

Preparation:

1. Preheat grill or grill pan.

2. Season the turkey breast fillets with olive oil, dried thyme, salt, and pepper.

3. Grill the turkey for 15-20 minutes, or until it is thoroughly cooked.

4. Boil the sweet potatoes until cooked, then mash them with a fork.

5. Steam the asparagus until crisp-tender.

6. Serve the grilled turkey on a bed of sweet potato mash, with asparagus on the side.

7. Garnish with fresh parsley.

Servings: Two.

Nutritional content: lean protein from turkey, complex carbohydrates from sweet potatoes, and vitamins from asparagus.

Miso Glazed Salmon with Brown Rice and Steamed Broccoli

Ingredients:

-2 salmon fillets

- 2 tablespoons miso paste

- 1 tablespoon soy sauce, and 1 tablespoon maple syrup.

- One cup of cooked brown rice.

- Two cups of broccoli florets

- Sesame seeds as garnish

- Sliced green onions as garnish

Preparation:

1. Preheat oven to 400°F (200°C).

2. In a mixing bowl, combine miso paste, soy sauce, and maple syrup to make the glaze.

3. Brush the salmon fillets with miso glaze.

4. Bake the salmon in the oven for 15-20 minutes, or until thoroughly done.

5. Steam the broccoli until soft.

6. Serve the salmon over brown rice, with steamed broccoli on the side.

7. Sprinkle with sesame seeds and sliced green onions.

Servings: Two.

Nutritional contents: omega-3 from salmon, balanced carbohydrates from brown rice, and vitamins from broccoli.

Quinoa-Black Bean Stuffed Bell Peppers with Avocado Salsa

Ingredients:

- 4 bell peppers, halved and seeds removed

- 1 cup quinoa, cooked

- 1 can (15 oz) black beans, drained and rinsed

- One cup of corn kernels

- Mix in 1 teaspoon cumin and 1 teaspoon chili powder.

- Season with salt and pepper to taste. - Make avocado salsa with tomatoes, red onion, and cilantro.

Preparation:

1. Preheat your oven to 375°F (190°C).

2. In a bowl, combine the quinoa, black beans, corn, cumin, chili powder, salt, and pepper.

3. Stuff bell pepper halves with quinoa mixture.

4. Bake for 25-30 minutes, until the peppers are soft.

5. Finish with avocado salsa before serving.

Serves: 4

Nutritional Contents: - Quinoa and black beans provide high fiber and protein, while bell peppers and avocado include vitamins.

Lemon and Honey Glazed Chicken Thighs with Cauliflower Mash

Ingredients:

- 4 chicken thighs (bone-in, skin-on)

- 2 tablespoons olive oil - 2 teaspoons honey

- Zest and juice from 1 lemon

- Add salt and pepper to taste.

- Chop one head of cauliflower. - Mince two cloves of garlic.

- 1/4 cup unsweetened almond milk.

- Fresh parsley as garnish

Preparation:

1. Preheat oven to 400°F (200°C).

2. In a mixing bowl, combine olive oil, honey, lemon zest, and lemon juice to make the glaze.

3. Season the chicken thighs with salt and pepper, then coat with the lemon-honey glaze.

4. Bake chicken in the oven for 30-35 minutes, or until thoroughly done.

5. Steam the cauliflower until tender, then mash with almond milk and minced garlic.

6. Serve chicken thighs with cauliflower mash.

7. Garnish with fresh parsley.

Serves: 4

Nutritional Contents: - Chicken thighs provide protein, cauliflower mash is low in carbs, and honey and lemon add natural sweetness.

Vegetable Stir-Fry with Turmeric Spiced Brown Rice

Ingredients:

- 2 cups chopped vegetables (broccoli florets, bell peppers, snap peas, carrots)

- 1 thinly sliced onion - 2 minced garlic cloves

- 1 tablespoon ginger, shredded

- 2 teaspoons of soy sauce (low sodium if desired)

- Use 1 tablespoon sesame oil and 1 tablespoon olive oil.

- Add salt and pepper to taste. - Garnish with sesame seeds.

- Green onions, cut for garnish.

For the turmeric-spiced brown rice:

- 1 cup brown rice

- 2 cups vegetable broth, and 1 teaspoon turmeric powder.

- Add salt to taste.

Preparation:

Turmeric Spiced Brown Rice:

1. In a pot, combine the brown rice, vegetable broth, turmeric powder, and salt.

2. Bring to a boil, then reduce heat, cover, and simmer until rice is cooked and liquid has been absorbed (per package directions).

3. Fluff rice with a fork, then set aside.

Vegetable Stir-fry:

1. Heat the olive oil in a large wok or skillet over medium-high heat.

2. Add the cut onions and simmer until tender.

3. Add the minced garlic and grated ginger, simmering for another 1-2 minutes until aromatic.

4. Add chopped mixed veggies to the wok and stir-fry until tender-crisp.

5. In a small bowl, combine the soy sauce and sesame oil. Pour over the vegetables and stir until evenly coated.

6. Add salt and pepper to taste.

7. Stir-fry the vegetables until they are thoroughly cooked yet still vivid.

8. Pour the veggie stir-fry over the turmeric-seasoned brown rice.

9. Sprinkle with sesame seeds and sliced green onions.

Serves: 4

Nutritional Contents: - Mixed vegetables provide vitamins and minerals, turmeric has anti-inflammatory properties, and the flavors are nutritious.

Snacks and Beverages for Healing

Anti-inflammatory Berry Bliss Smoothie

Ingredients:

- One cup of mixed berries (blueberries, strawberries, raspberries)

- One-half banana

- One cup of spinach leaves.

- One spoonful of chia seeds

- Half cup Greek yogurt

- One cup of almond milk.

- Ice cubes (Optional)

- Honey for sweetness is optional.

Preparation:

1. Blend mixed berries, banana, spinach, chia seeds, Greek yogurt, and almond milk.

2. Blend until smooth.

3. If desired, add more ice cubes and combine again.

4. If needed, sweeten with honey.

5. Pour into a glass and enjoy the anti-inflammatory properties of the Berry Bliss smoothie.

Serves: 1

Nutritional Contents: - High in antioxidants from berries, omega-3 from chia seeds, and vitamins from banana and spinach.

Turmeric-infused Golden Milk Elixir.

Ingredients:

- 1 cup almond milk

- 1 teaspoon turmeric powder.

-1/2 teaspoon cinnamon

- One-quarter teaspoon of ginger powder

- Add a pinch of black pepper, 1 teaspoon of honey, and 1/2 teaspoon coconut oil (optional).

Preparation:

1. Heat almond milk in a small saucepan on medium heat.

2. Combine the turmeric, cinnamon, ginger, black pepper, and honey.

3. Whisk until well blended and hot.

4. If preferred, add the coconut oil and stir until it melts.

5. Pour into a mug and sip the calming golden milk elixir.

Serves: 1

Nutritional benefits: turmeric's anti-inflammatory properties, warming spices, and honey for sweetness.

Healing Green Tea Infusion with Ginger and Mint

Ingredients:

- One green tea bag.

-1-inch sliced ginger

- fresh mint leaves

- 1 tablespoon honey, and optional lemon slices for garnish.

Preparation:

1. Steep the green tea bag in boiling water per package instructions.

2. Incorporate sliced ginger and fresh mint leaves into the tea.

3. Let the flavors infuse for a few minutes.

4. Stir in the honey until it's dissolved.

5. Garnish with lemon slices if desired.

6. Strain and serve the therapeutic green tea infusion.

Serves: 1

Nutritional Contents: - Green tea contains antioxidants, ginger and mint have calming effects, and honey provides natural sweetness.

Nutrient-dense Avocado and Salmon Sushi Rolls

Ingredients:

- Nori seaweed sheets.

- Cook 1 cup sushi rice and season with rice vinegar. - Slice 1/2 avocado.

- Two ounces of smoked salmon

- Cucumber strips.

- Soy sauce and wasabi for dipping.

Preparation:

1. Set a nori sheet on a bamboo sushi mat.

2. Spread a thin layer of seasoned sushi rice over the nori.

3. Arrange avocado slices, smoked salmon, and cucumber strips on one side of the rice.

4. Roll the nori tightly using the sushi rolling mat.

5. Use a little water to seal the edge.

6. Cut the roll into bite-size pieces.

7. Serve with soy sauce and wasabi.

Servings: 2

Nutritional Contents: - Avocado and salmon provide healthy fats and omega-3 fatty acids, with a pleasing flavor profile.

Quinoa Power Bowl and Roasted Vegetables

Ingredients:

Ingredients:

-1 cup cooked quinoa

- roasted veggies (sweet potatoes, bell peppers, zucchini)

- halved cherry tomatoes, and 1/4 cup crumbled feta cheese.

- A handful of baby spinach leaves.

- For the dressing, use olive oil and balsamic vinegar. –Add salt and pepper to taste.

Preparation:

1. Cook the quinoa according to the package instructions.

2. Roast various vegetables in olive oil till soft.

3. In a bowl, combine the quinoa, roasted veggies, cherry tomatoes, feta cheese, and spinach.

4. Finish with a drizzle of olive oil and balsamic vinegar.

5. Add salt and pepper to taste.

Servings: Two.

Nutritional Contents: - Quinoa provides high protein and fiber, vegetables provide vitamins, and olive oil and feta contain healthy fats.

Pain Relief Trail Mix with Nuts and Anti-Inflammatory Spices

Ingredients:

- 1/2 cup almonds

- 1/2 cup walnuts.

-1/4 cup pumpkin seeds

- 1/4 cup dried tart cherries.

- Use 1 teaspoon turmeric and 1/2 teaspoon cinnamon.

- Add a pinch of cayenne pepper and 1 tablespoon of honey.

Preparation:

1. In a bowl, combine the almonds, walnuts, pumpkin seeds, and dried cherries.

2. In a small bowl, combine the turmeric, cinnamon, cayenne pepper, and honey.

3. Toss the nuts and fruit with the spice mixture.

4. Spread the mixture onto a baking sheet and bake at 350°F (175°C) for 10-15 minutes, or until lightly browned.

5. Let it cool before storing in an airtight container.

Servings: 2.

Nutritional contents: Nuts and seeds include omega-3 fatty acids, while turmeric and cinnamon have anti-inflammatory effects.

Ginger and Lemon Chia Seed Pudding

Ingredients:

-1/4 cup chia seeds.

- 1 cup almond milk

- 1 tablespoon grated fresh ginger, and 1 lemon zest and juice.

- 1 tablespoon of honey and sliced strawberries for topping.

Preparation:

1. combine chia seeds, almond milk, ginger, lemon zest, lemon juice, and honey in a mixing dish.

2. Stir well and chill for at least 4 hours or overnight to thicken.

3. Before serving, garnish with cut strawberries.

Serves: 1

Nutritional Contents: - Chia seeds contain omega-3 fatty acids, ginger and lemon provide calming effects, and honey provides natural sweetness.

Soothing Sweet Potato and Carrot Soup.

Ingredients:

- 2 peeled and diced sweet potatoes

- 3 peeled and sliced carrots

- 1 chopped onion - 2 minced garlic cloves

- 1 grated fresh ginger

- 4 cups vegetable broth

- 1/2 teaspoon turmeric powder.

- Season with salt and pepper to taste.

- Add coconut milk for richness (optional).

Preparation:

1. Cook onion, garlic, and ginger in a saucepan until softened.

2. Combine the chopped sweet potatoes, carrots, turmeric powder, and vegetable broth.

3. Simmer until the vegetables are soft.

4. Using an immersion blender, or transferring to a blender, blend until smooth.

5. Add salt and pepper to taste.

6. If preferred, add coconut milk for an additional creamy texture.

Serves: 4

Nutritional Contents: - Sweet potatoes and carrots provide vitamins and fiber, while turmeric has anti-inflammatory properties.

Grilled pineapple and chicken skewers with a turmeric marinade.

Ingredients:

For the turmeric marinade:

- 1/4 cup olive oil and 1 teaspoon turmeric powder.

- Incorporate 1 teaspoon cumin and 1 teaspoon paprika.

- 2 garlic cloves, minced

- Add salt and pepper to taste.

For the skewers:

- 1 pound of chicken breast, cubed

- One fresh pineapple, peeled and cut into chunks

- Soak wooden skewers in a bowl of water for 30 min.

Preparation:

Turmeric marinade:

1. In a bowl, combine the olive oil, turmeric powder, cumin, paprika, minced garlic, salt, and pepper.

Skewers:

1. Marinate the chicken cubes in the turmeric marinade for at least 30 minutes in the fridge.

2. Preheat your grill or grill pan.

3. Thread the marinated chicken and pineapple slices on the soaked skewers.

4. Grill the skewers for 10-15 minutes, rotating occasionally, until the chicken is fully cooked and the pineapple is caramelized.

5. Serve immediately.

Serves: 4

Nutritional Contents: - Chicken provides lean protein, turmeric has anti-inflammatory properties, and grilled pineapple adds natural sweetness.

Dark Chocolate and Almond Butter Energy Bites

Ingredients:

-1 cup old-fashioned oats and 1/2 cup almond butter.

- Add 1/3 cup honey and 1/2 cup dark chocolate chips.

- Combine 1/2 cup ground flaxseed

-1 teaspoon vanilla essence, and a pinch of salt.

Preparation:

1. In a bowl, combine the oats, almond butter, honey, dark chocolate chips, ground flaxseed, vanilla essence, and a pinch of salt.

2. Refrigerate the mixture for 30 minutes until solid.

3. Once cooled, use your hands to form the dough into bite-sized balls.

4. Keep in an airtight jar in the fridge.

Servings: Approximately 20 energy nibbles.

Nutritional Contents: - Almond butter provides protein and healthy fats, while oats and flaxseed provide fiber. Honey and dark chocolate add sweetness.

CHAPTER 4

Cooking Techniques and Tips.

For people dealing with fibromyalgia, the kitchen may be a source of comfort and empowerment. Adopting cooking practices that promote nutrient retention, as well as advice for speedy, painless meal preparation, can make the culinary journey both nourishing and pleasant.

Cooking Techniques that Preserve Nutrients

Choosing cooking methods that preserve the nutritional worth of ingredients is critical for fibromyalgia patients.

Steaming, a mild cooking method, ensures that veggies retain their bright colors and nutrients. It is a simple yet efficient method for preserving the nutritional value of broccoli, carrots, and other fibrous vegetables.

Roasting, especially for root vegetables, increases taste while preserving nutritional value. Tossing veggies like sweet potatoes and beets in a little coat of olive oil and roasting them yields a tasty side dish while preserving nutrition.

Poaching is another technique for carefully cooking meats like fish or poultry without exposing them to high temperatures. This approach not only keeps moisture but also protects the nutritious value of the protein.

Tips for Effective and Painless Meal Preparation

Efficient meal preparation can make a significant difference for people suffering from fibromyalgia-related fatigue and pain.

Batch cooking becomes a useful tool, allowing for the creation of bigger amounts of meals that may be saved for later use.

This reduces the frequency of strenuous cooking sessions while ensuring a consistent supply of healthful foods.

Investing in kitchen gadgets that make the job easier, such as a food processor for chopping and a slow cooker for hands-free cooking, can greatly minimize the physical strain associated with meal preparation.

Pre-cut vegetables and pre-packaged, healthful products can save time and make meal preparation easier and less painful.

Breaking down the meal preparation process into smaller, more manageable steps can make a significant difference.

For example, cutting vegetables ahead of time or marinating proteins ahead of time allows for more efficient cooking sessions by dispersing the task across multiple days.

Strategic kitchen organization, such as keeping frequently used goods within easy reach, can help to eliminate unnecessary movement and strain. Adopting a comfortable standing or sitting position while preparing ingredients can also help to ensure a pain-free cooking experience.

Lifestyle Strategies outside the Kitchen

While the kitchen is important in controlling fibromyalgia, holistic well-being includes lifestyle measures that go beyond culinary choices.

Incorporating exercise for physical healing, implementing stress management techniques, and prioritizing sleep hygiene become critical components in the route to fibromyalgia alleviation.

Exercise, when adjusted to individual capacities, can be an effective technique for physical rehabilitation in the treatment of fibromyalgia.

Walking, swimming, and mild yoga are all low-impact activities that can help you increase your flexibility, reduce muscular stiffness, and feel better overall.

Consistency is essential, and individuals should begin with short sessions and progressively increase duration as tolerance increases.

Engaging in enjoyable activities, such as dance, tai chi, or water aerobics, not only enhances physical recuperation but also improves mental and emotional health.

20 Home Exercise Ideas

1. Gentle Stretching:

- Begin gently stretching in a comfortable seated or standing position.

- Begin with gradual, controlled neck stretches that move gently in several directions.

- Gradually expand the stretches to incorporate the arms, shoulders, and legs.

- Hold each stretch for 15-30 seconds, avoiding any painful movements.

- Repeat the stretching practice 5-10 times, changing the intensity based on personal comfort levels.

2. Neck Stretches:

- Sit or stand with a straight spine and relaxed shoulders.

- Slowly tilt your head to the side, bringing your ear close to your shoulder.

- Hold the stretch for 15 to 30 seconds, feeling a mild pull along the side of your neck.

- Repeat on the opposite side.

- Repeat 5-10 times, progressively increasing range of motion based on comfort.

3. Shoulder Rolls:

- Sit or stand comfortably, arms hanging loosely by sides.

- Raise your shoulders to your ears and then roll them back in a circular motion.

- Repeat the shoulder roll for 10-15 seconds, then reverse direction.

- Perform 2-3 sets of smooth, controlled motions.

- To avoid tension, do not elevate your shoulders too high.

4. Arm Circles:

- Stand with feet shoulder-width apart and extend arms to sides.

- Start forming little circles with your arms and progressively increase the size.

- After 15–30 seconds, reverse the orientation of the circles.

- Perform 2-3 sets with fluid and controlled motions.

- Adjust the circle size to your comfort level.

5. Seated Leg Lifts:

- Sit comfortably in a chair, back straight, feet flat on the floor.

- Lift one leg straight out in front and hold for a few seconds.

- Slowly lower the leg back down, avoiding any sudden movements.

- Repeat for the opposite leg.

- Do 10-15 repetitions each leg, progressively increasing as tolerated.

6. Ankle Rotations:

- Sit or lie comfortably.

- Lift one foot off the ground, then rotate the ankle clockwise for 15-30 seconds.

- Reverse the direction and rotate the ankle counterclockwise.

- Switch to the opposite ankle and repeat the rotations.

- Do 2-3 sets per ankle, concentrating on smooth, controlled rotations.

7. Water Aerobics:

- Use a pool with a comfortable temperature.

- Practice low-impact aerobic workouts like water walking, leg lifts, and arm movements.

- Move carefully and with control to reduce joint tension.

- Start with 20-30 minutes of water aerobics and progressively increase the duration as your fitness improves.

- Pay attention to individual energy levels and adjust exercises accordingly.

8. Walking:

- Use a flat, even surface for walking.

Start at a leisurely and comfortable speed.

- Concentrate on keeping proper posture and a natural stride.

- Start with a modest period, like 10 minutes, and progressively expand over time.

- Pay attention to your body, modifying the pace and distance to suit your energy level and comfort.

9. Tai Chi:

- Choose a calm and comfortable area with enough space to move around.

- To find your center, start with deep, relaxed breathing.

- Concentrate on balance and coordination while moving gently and fluidly through the Tai Chi form.

- Practice a series of Tai Chi forms or movements, focusing on slow and controlled motions.

- Practice for 15-30 minutes, progressively increasing the time as stamina develops.

10. Yoga:

- Choose a yoga regimen that focuses on soft positions and attentive breathing.

- Begin with a brief meditation or relaxation technique to concentrate your mind.

- Continue through a sequence of yoga poses that emphasize flexibility and balance.

- Hold each pose for 15-30 seconds, inhaling deeply and at a moderate pace.

- Finish the routine with a short relaxation or meditation session.

11. Deep Breathing Exercises: - Choose a quiet and comfortable location to sit or lie down.

- Inhale deeply through your nose, expanding your lungs completely.

- Exhale slowly through pursed lips to relieve tension and promote relaxation.

- Practice diaphragmatic breathing, allowing your belly to rise and fall with each breath.

- Practice deep breathing for 5-10 minutes, progressively increasing the duration as you feel comfortable.

12. Stationary Cycling: - Place a stationary bike in a comfortable and well-ventilated place.

- Begin with low resistance and a leisurely speed.

- Pedal steadily for 15-20 minutes while maintaining a smooth and steady rhythm.

- Gradually increase resistance and time based on your comfort level.

- Maintain proper posture and avoid putting excessive strain on your joints.

13. Chair Exercises:

- Sit comfortably on a firm chair, feet flat on the ground.

- Start with seated marches, raising one knee at a time.

- Progress to sitting leg extensions by straightening one leg at a time.

- Incorporate seated torso twists and side bends to improve flexibility.

- Do 10-15 reps of each exercise, gradually increasing as tolerated.

14. Pilates:

-Begin on a mat or padded surface.

- Concentrate on calm, flowing motions that activate the core.

- Include Pilates movements such as leg circles, the hundred, and planks.

- Focus on good form and alignment during each action.

- Perform a Pilates routine for 20-30 minutes, modifying the intensity based on your needs.

15. Wall Push-ups:

- Stand facing a wall, feet hip-width apart.

- Position your hands shoulder-high on the wall.

- Do push-ups with your elbows bent and your chest against the wall.

- Maintain a straight posture while engaging your core.

- Repeat 10-15 times, progressively increasing as strength develops.

16. Balance Exercises:

- Use a strong surface for support if necessary.

- Lift one foot off the ground while maintaining balance with the other.

- Hold the pose for 15-30 seconds, focusing on stability.

- Change to the other leg and repeat.

- Gradually go to increasingly difficult activities such as heel-to-toe walking or single-leg standing, adapting the difficulty to suit individual comfort.

17. Gentle Strength Training:

- Start with light resistance, like resistance bands or light weights.

- Concentrate on the primary muscle groups, which include the arms, legs, and core.

- Exercises include bicep curls, leg lifts, and sitting leg presses.

- Begin with 1-2 sets of 10-15 repetitions per exercise, progressively increasing the intensity as tolerated.

- Pay attention to the appropriate form and avoid over-exertion.

18. Mind-Body Connection:

- Find a quiet location and sit or lie comfortably.

- Use mindfulness meditation or guided visualization to strengthen the mind-body connection.

- Concentrate on your breathing, sensations in your body, and positive affirmations.

- Practice these exercises for 10-15 minutes each day, progressively extending the duration as your mindfulness skills improve.

19. Self-Massage:

- Apply gentle circular motions using fingertips or a massage instrument.

- Concentrate on areas with muscle tension or soreness, such as the neck, shoulders, and back.

- Adjust pressure according to your comfort, avoiding excessive force.

- Incorporate 5-10 minutes of self-massage into your daily regimen, with a focus on areas of difficulty.

20. Warm Water Pool Exercises:

- Choose a pool with a reasonable temperature.

- Practice low-impact activities including leg lifts, arm circles, and slow water walking. Use water's buoyancy to lessen the impact on joints.

- Aim for 20-30 minutes of pool exercises, progressively increasing the intensity and duration as your fitness increases.

- Pay attention to individual energy levels and adjust exercises accordingly.

Remember that people with fibromyalgia should start carefully, listen to their bodies, and advance gradually. A consultation with a healthcare practitioner is required to develop a safe and effective workout regimen based on individual needs and restrictions.

Stress Management Techniques

Fibromyalgia and stress frequently coexist, resulting in a vicious cycle of worsening symptoms. Implementing stress management practices is critical for breaking the pattern.

Mindfulness activities, such as meditation and deep breathing exercises, create a mental sanctuary, promoting calm and reducing stress.

Hobbies, such as reading, painting, and gardening, provide a welcome distraction and opportunity for creative expression.

Setting realistic goals and boundaries, both at work and in personal life, helps to manage stress and avoid overload.

Connecting with a support system, whether it's friends, family, or a support group, provides emotional outlets and fosters a sense of community. These measures all help to reduce stress, resulting in a more resilient foundation for fibromyalgia management.

Sleep Hygiene and Fibromyalgia Relief

Quality sleep is essential for fibromyalgia alleviation, and correct sleep hygiene practices become critical.

Establishing a consistent sleep pattern, which includes going to bed and waking up at the same time every day, aids in regulating the body's internal clock and enhances sleep quality.

Creating a good sleep environment entails optimizing variables such as room temperature, lighting, and mattress comfort. Minimizing screen time before bed and establishing soothing evening rituals, such as reading or gentle stretching, communicate to the body that it is time to unwind.

Limiting caffeine and alcohol intake, especially in the evening, promotes better sleep. Regular physical activity earlier in the day increases general weariness and promotes a more restful night's sleep.

Lifestyle practices outside of the kitchen are critical components of fibromyalgia management. Individuals can create a holistic approach to well-being that extends far beyond the kitchen by including exercise for physical recovery, implementing stress management techniques, and emphasizing sleep hygiene.

Community and Support

In the rich fabric of fibromyalgia management, community and support shine as beacons of understanding and shared strength.

Connecting with those facing similar struggles and embracing the opportunity to share one's story while learning from others become pillars of support on the path to fibromyalgia relief.

Connecting With Others Managing Fibromyalgia

Isolation may be a difficult foe when dealing with fibromyalgia, and connecting with others who understand the complexities of the condition can provide solace and empowerment. Online forums, support groups, and local fibromyalgia meet-ups provide an opportunity to share experiences, exchange insights, and develop a feeling of community.

Engaging with others who have similar challenges not only provides emotional support but also practical advice and coping skills. Knowing that one is not alone in facing the problems of fibromyalgia can be a transforming experience, forming a network of understanding that extends beyond the condition's restrictions.

Sharing Your Journey and Learning from Others

Sharing one's fibromyalgia journey is not only a vulnerable act, but it also makes a significant addition to the community's collective knowledge pool. Individuals share insights into their personal experiences, struggles, and achievements, which may resonate with others and generate a sense of unity.

In contrast, learning from the experiences of other community members provides a plethora of information and various viewpoints. Each person's experience with fibromyalgia is unique, and the collective wisdom acquired from shared stories can open up new paths of coping symptom management, and lifestyle changes.

Individuals can participate in support groups or online communities to ask concerns, seek advice, and encourage others who are facing similar issues. The sharing of knowledge becomes reciprocal, resulting in a dynamic ecosystem in which everyone contributes to and benefits from the community's collective wisdom.

When people connect with others who have fibromyalgia, they develop a supportive network that not only understands their challenges but also serves as a platform for sharing, learning, and growing together on the path to relief and well-being.

CHAPTER 5

Meal Plans for Fibromyalgia Relief

Navigating the problems of fibromyalgia requires not only individual items but also the careful planning of meal plans that are tailored specifically to pain management.

Weekly food planning becomes a strategic and empowering tool for people looking for relief from fibromyalgia's persistent symptoms.

Weekly Meal Plans for Pain Management.

Creating meal plans for fibromyalgia alleviation requires a careful selection of ingredients known for their anti-inflammatory and nutritious characteristics.

Begin the week with a colorful and antioxidant-rich mixed berry and spinach smoothie for breakfast, setting a positive tone for the day.

Lunches could contain grilled salmon with omega-3 fatty acids and a quinoa salad filled with vibrant veggies.

Anti-inflammatory spices such as turmeric and ginger can be used in dinner recipes like vegetable curry or lean protein stir-fry to bring flavor as well as therapeutic benefits.

Snacks can be a delicious combination of nuts and seeds, delivering not only a pleasing crunch but also important nutrients. Choosing nutrient-dense snacks throughout the day will help you maintain your energy levels and manage fibromyalgia-related fatigue.

Adjusting Diets for Different Symptom Intensity

Recognizing the dynamic nature of fibromyalgia symptoms is essential for tailoring meal plans to different levels of intensity.

On days when exhaustion is severe, simpler food options that need little preparation can be used. This could include simple soups, fruit-flavored yogurt, or whole-grain crackers with hummus.In contrast, during times of intense pain, anti-inflammatory substances such as ginger and turmeric can take center stage in meal planning.

Comforting yet nourishing meals, such as a sweet potato and lentil stew or a baked salmon fillet with roasted veggies, can provide both relief and support.

Hydration is key in fibromyalgia management, so meal planning should include herbal teas, infused water, or hydration soups. These liquid solutions not only improve general health but also help to maintain hydration levels, which is often forgotten when managing fibromyalgia symptoms.

In essence, fibromyalgia meal plans become dynamic tools that may be altered in response to the ebb and flow of symptoms. Individuals can build a sustainable and pleasurable approach to fibromyalgia management through their regular meals by incorporating a variety of nutrient-dense foods, and anti-inflammatory substances, and adapting to the severity of symptoms.

21-DAY MEAL PLAN

Week 1:

Day 1

Breakfast: Turmeric Infused Quinoa Breakfast Bowl

Lunch: Anti-Inflammatory Turmeric Chicken Salad

Dinner: Turmeric Infused Quinoa Bowl with Roasted Vegetables

Snack: Anti-Inflammatory Berry Bliss Smoothie

Day 2

Breakfast: Omega-3 Packed Chia Seed Pudding with Berries

Lunch: Omega-3 Packed Salmon Power Bowl

Dinner: Salmon and Avocado Citrus Salad with Mixed Greens

Snack: Turmeric-infused Golden Milk Elixir

Day 3

Breakfast: Anti-Inflammatory Avocado Toast with Smoked Salmon

Lunch: Quinoa and Veggie Stuffed Bell Peppers

Dinner: Ginger-Turmeric Chicken Soup with Quinoa and Kale

Snack: Healing Green Tea Infusion with Ginger and Mint

Day 4

Breakfast: Protein-Packed Greek Yogurt Parfait with Almond Butter

Lunch: Ginger-Turmeric Carrot Soup

Dinner: Baked Cod with Lemon and Herb Quinoa Pilaf

Snack: Nutrient-packed Avocado and Salmon Sushi Rolls

Day 5

Breakfast: Spinach and Mushroom Egg White Omelette

Lunch: Avocado and Spinach Smoothie with Flaxseed

Dinner: Spinach and Chickpea Curry with Basmati Rice

Snack: Quinoa Power Bowl with Roasted Vegetables

Day 6

Breakfast: Fiber-Rich Oatmeal with Fresh Fruits and Nuts

Lunch: Mediterranean Chickpea Salad with Olive Oil Dressing

Dinner: Grilled Turkey Breast with Sweet Potato Mash and Asparagus

Snack: Pain-Relief Trail Mix with Nuts and Anti-Inflammatory Spices

Day 7

Breakfast: Salmon and Sweet Potato Hash with Turmeric

Lunch: Baked Sweet Potato with Cinnamon and Coconut Oil

Dinner: Miso-Glazed Salmon with Brown Rice and Steamed Broccoli

Snack: Ginger-Lemon Chia Seed Pudding

Week 2:

Breakfast: Berry Blast Chia Seed Pudding

Lunch: Quinoa and Veggie Stuffed Bell Peppers

Dinner: Quinoa and Black Bean Stuffed Bell Peppers with Avocado Salsa

Snack: Healing Green Tea Infusion with Ginger and Mint

Breakfast: Green Smoothie Bowl with Kale and Pineapple

Lunch: Baked Sweet Potato with Cinnamon and Coconut Oil

Dinner: Miso-Glazed Salmon with Brown Rice and Steamed Broccoli

Snack: Dark Chocolate and Almond Butter Energy Bites

Breakfast: Cinnamon Walnut Buckwheat Pancakes

Lunch: Mediterranean Chickpea Salad with Olive Oil Dressing

Dinner: Grilled Turkey Breast with Sweet Potato Mash and Asparagus

Snack: Ginger-Lemon Chia Seed Pudding

Day 11

Breakfast: Coconut Milk and Berry Quinoa Porridge

Lunch: Anti-Oxidant Rich Berry and Kale Smoothie

Dinner: Lemon-Honey Glazed Chicken Thighs with Cauliflower Mash

Snack: Soothing Sweet Potato and Carrot Soup

Day 12

Breakfast: Turmeric Infused Quinoa Breakfast Bowl

Lunch: Anti-Inflammatory Turmeric Chicken Salad

Dinner: Turmeric Infused Quinoa Bowl with Roasted Vegetables

Snack: Anti-Inflammatory Berry Bliss Smoothie

Day 13

Breakfast: Omega-3 Packed Chia Seed Pudding with Berries

Lunch: Omega-3 Packed Salmon Power Bowl

Dinner: Salmon and Avocado Citrus Salad with Mixed Greens

Snack: Turmeric-infused Golden Milk Elixir

Day 14

Breakfast: Anti-Inflammatory Avocado Toast with Smoked Salmon

Lunch: Quinoa and Veggie Stuffed Bell Peppers

Dinner: Ginger-Turmeric Chicken Soup with Quinoa and Kale

Snack: Healing Green Tea Infusion with Ginger and Mint

Day 15

Breakfast: Cinnamon Walnut Buckwheat Pancakes

Lunch: Green Tea Infused Quinoa Bowl with Grilled Chicken

Dinner: Quinoa and Black Bean Stuffed Bell Peppers with Avocado Salsa

Snack: Dark Chocolate and Almond Butter Energy Bites

Day 16

Breakfast: Coconut Milk and Berry Quinoa Porridge

Lunch: Anti-Oxidant Rich Berry and Kale Smoothie

Dinner: Lemon-Honey Glazed Chicken Thighs with Cauliflower Mash

Snack: Soothing Sweet Potato and Carrot Soup

Day 17

Breakfast: Turmeric Infused Quinoa Breakfast Bowl

Lunch: Anti-Inflammatory Turmeric Chicken Salad

Dinner: Turmeric Infused Quinoa Bowl with Roasted Vegetables

Snack: Anti-Inflammatory Berry Bliss Smoothie

Day 18

Breakfast: Omega-3 Packed Chia Seed Pudding with Berries

Lunch: Omega-3 Packed Salmon Power Bowl

Dinner: Salmon and Avocado Citrus Salad with Mixed Greens

Snack: Turmeric-infused Golden Milk Elixir

Day 19

Breakfast: Anti-Inflammatory Avocado Toast with Smoked Salmon

Lunch: Quinoa and Veggie Stuffed Bell Peppers

Dinner: Ginger-Turmeric Chicken Soup with Quinoa and Kale

Snack: Healing Green Tea Infusion with Ginger and Mint

Day 20

Breakfast: Protein-Packed Greek Yogurt Parfait with Almond Butter

Lunch: Ginger-Turmeric Carrot Soup

Dinner: Baked Cod with Lemon and Herb Quinoa Pilaf

Snack: Nutrient-packed Avocado and Salmon Sushi Rolls

Day 21

Breakfast: Spinach and Mushroom Egg White Omelette

Lunch: Avocado and Spinach Smoothie with Flaxseed

Dinner: Spinach and Chickpea Curry with Basmati Rice

Snack: Quinoa Power Bowl with Roasted Vegetables

Conclusion

As we come to the end of the "Fibromyalgia Cookbook," we find ourselves at the confluence of culinary inquiry and well-being.

This book was written with the premise that controlling fibromyalgia is a multifaceted task, and the kitchen serves as a sanctuary where therapeutic ingredients and mindful culinary skills can coexist.

In these chapters, we've looked at the dietary foundations that support fibromyalgia alleviation, celebrated the power of anti-inflammatory substances, and created practical meal plans to ease pain and exhaustion.

Cooking techniques aimed at nutrition retention have changed the kitchen into a place of empowerment, where efficiency and convenience reign.

We've broadened our journey beyond the culinary arena, investigating lifestyle techniques, developing relationships within a supportive group, and acknowledging that the path to relief is paved with patience, adaptation, and the celebration of modest wins.

This cookbook is more than just a compilation of recipes; it's a companion on your journey to wellness.

It encourages you to eat a well-balanced and tasty diet rich in the healing properties of nature's bounty. Every recipe, from anti-inflammatory spices to nutrient-dense meals, is a step toward not only managing but also living with fibromyalgia.

As you close the book and walk into your kitchen, may the aromas of healing herbs and the sizzle of nourishing ingredients bring you joy and strength.

May each meal you cook be an act of self-care, a nutritious gift for your body and spirit. Remember that this is not a voyage of perfection, but rather of progress, adaptation, and self-discovery.

The "Fibromyalgia Cookbook" invites you to experience the flavors of empowerment, serving as a culinary guide to turning fibromyalgia obstacles into chances for recovery.

Whether you're attempting a new dish, sharing your experiences with others, or simply finding comfort in the kitchen, may this book inspire, encourage, and provide delightful moments on your journey to well-being.

Here's to enjoying the nutritious path ahead, filled with the warmth of supportive groups, the healing power of ingredients, and the inner strength that comes from within.

Bon appétit, and happy cooking!